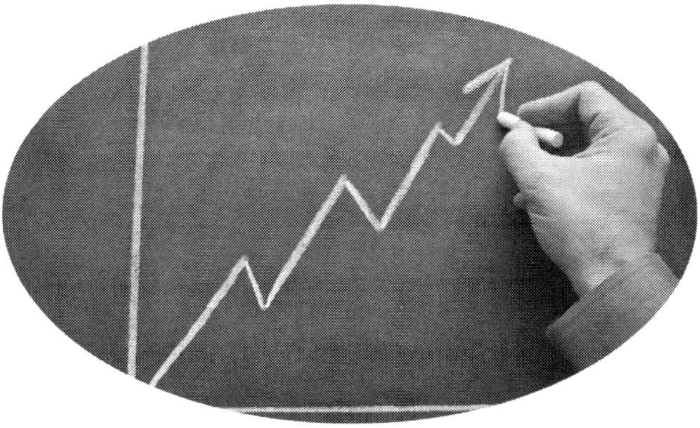

LET'S DO THIS

SUCCESS LOG

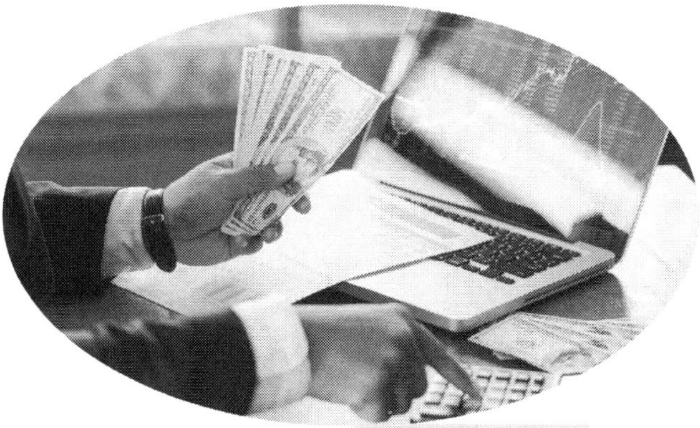

CABANA PUBLISHING

CABANA
PUBLISHING, LLC

CONGRATS

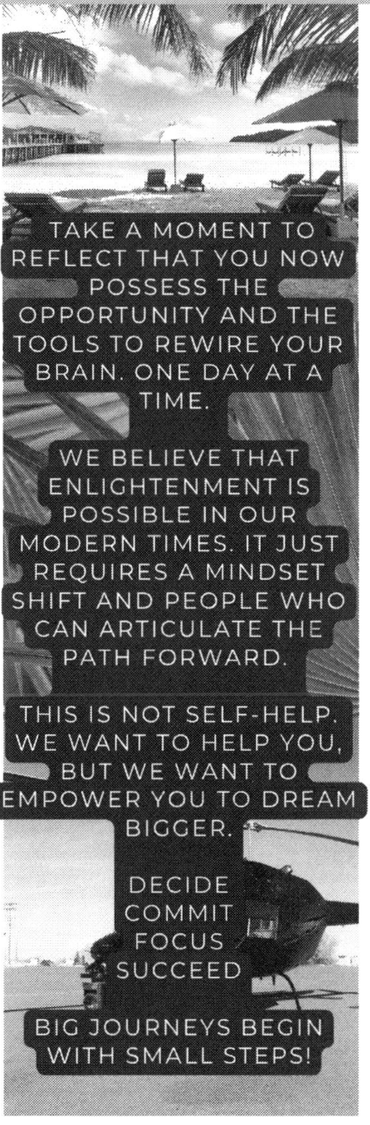
TAKE A MOMENT TO REFLECT THAT YOU NOW POSSESS THE OPPORTUNITY AND THE TOOLS TO REWIRE YOUR BRAIN. ONE DAY AT A TIME.
WE BELIEVE THAT ENLIGHTENMENT IS POSSIBLE IN OUR MODERN TIMES. IT JUST REQUIRES A MINDSET SHIFT AND PEOPLE WHO CAN ARTICULATE THE PATH FORWARD.
THIS IS NOT SELF-HELP. WE WANT TO HELP YOU, BUT WE WANT TO EMPOWER YOU TO DREAM BIGGER.
DECIDE
COMMIT
FOCUS
SUCCEED
BIG JOURNEYS BEGIN WITH SMALL STEPS!

3 STEP

PROCESS

INTROSPECTION

SELF-AWARENESS IS THE FIRST STEP TO IMPROVE. WHAT IS WORKING? WHAT ISN'T WORKING? WHAT ARE YOUR INTENTIONS? WHAT ARE YOUR GOALS? WHERE DO YOU NEED TO FOCUS?

DAY

BUDDHA SAID THE SECRET TO YOUR FUTURE IS IN YOUR DAILY ROUTINE. JRR TOLKIEN SAID THAT LITTLE BY LITTLE ONE TRAVELS FAR. MAP OUT YOUR DAY FOR SUCCESS

NIGHT

HOW DID YOU DO? WHAT DID YOU DO RIGHT? WHAT CAN BE DONE DIFFERENTLY? WHAT DID YOU LEARN?

LIFE

GOALS

FOR EACH OF THE CATEGORIES BELOW, WRITE DOWN THINGS YOU ARE DOING WELL AND WHERE YOU NEED IMPROVEMENT. TAKE THE TIME TO REFLECT ON THESE, AND WRITE A GOAL FOR EACH CATEGORY.

CATEGORY	WHAT I'M DOING WELL	WHERE I NEED IMPROVEMENT	MY GOALS
FAMILY			
FRIENDS			
WORK/ SCHOOL			
BODY			
MENTAL HEALTH			
SPIRITUALITY			

LIFE

GOALS

FOR EACH OF THE CATEGORIES BELOW, WRITE DOWN THINGS YOU ARE DOING WELL AND WHERE YOU NEED IMPROVEMENT. TAKE THE TIME TO REFLECT ON THESE, AND WRITE A GOAL FOR EACH CATEGORY.

CATEGORY	WHAT I'M DOING WELL	WHERE I NEED IMPROVEMENT	MY GOALS
FAMILY			
FRIENDS			
WORK/ SCHOOL			
BODY			
MENTAL HEALTH			
SPIRITUALITY			

UNDERSTANDING

GOALS

ACHIEVING OUR GOALS IS DEPENDENT ON WHETHER WE TAKE ACTION.
USE THE TABLE BELOW TO UNDERSTAND THE "WHY" OF YOUR GOALS.

GOAL:

WHAT WILL THIS GIVE YOU?

AND WHAT WILL THIS GIVE YOU?

AND WHAT WILL THIS GIVE YOU?

AND WHAT WILL THIS GIVE YOU?

SO, WHY IS THIS GOAL IMPORTANT?

UNDERSTANDING

GOALS

ACHIEVING OUR GOALS IS DEPENDENT ON WHETHER WE TAKE ACTION.
USE THE TABLE BELOW TO UNDERSTAND THE "WHY" OF YOUR GOALS.

GOAL:

WHAT WILL THIS GIVE YOU?

AND WHAT WILL THIS GIVE YOU?

AND WHAT WILL THIS GIVE YOU?

AND WHAT WILL THIS GIVE YOU?

SO, WHY IS THIS GOAL IMPORTANT?

UNDERSTANDING

GOALS

ACHIEVING OUR GOALS IS DEPENDENT ON WHETHER WE TAKE ACTION. USE THE TABLE BELOW TO UNDERSTAND THE "WHY" OF YOUR GOALS.

GOAL:

WHAT WILL THIS GIVE YOU?

AND WHAT WILL THIS GIVE YOU?

AND WHAT WILL THIS GIVE YOU?

AND WHAT WILL THIS GIVE YOU?

SO, WHY IS THIS GOAL IMPORTANT?

UNDERSTANDING

GOALS

ACHIEVING OUR GOALS IS DEPENDENT ON WHETHER WE TAKE ACTION. USE THE TABLE BELOW TO UNDERSTAND THE "WHY" OF YOUR GOALS.

GOAL:

WHAT WILL THIS GIVE YOU?

AND WHAT WILL THIS GIVE YOU?

AND WHAT WILL THIS GIVE YOU?

AND WHAT WILL THIS GIVE YOU?

SO, WHY IS THIS GOAL IMPORTANT?

SMART

GOALS

WHEN SETTING GOALS, MAKE SURE IT FOLLOWS THE SMART STRUCTURE. USE THE QUESTIONS BELOW TO CREATE YOUR GOALS.

S	SPECIFIC WHAT DO I WANT TO ACCOMPLISH?	
M	MEASURABLE HOW WILL I KNOW WHEN IT IS ACCOMPLISHED?	
A	ACHIEVABLE HOW CAN THE GOAL BE ACCOMPLISHED?	
R	RELEVANT DOES THIS SEEM WORTHWHILE?	
T	TIME BOUND WHEN CAN I ACCOMPLISH THIS GOAL?	

SMART

GOALS

WHEN SETTING GOALS, MAKE SURE IT FOLLOWS THE SMART STRUCTURE. USE THE QUESTIONS BELOW TO CREATE YOUR GOALS.

S	SPECIFIC WHAT DO I WANT TO ACCOMPLISH?	
M	MEASURABLE HOW WILL I KNOW WHEN IT IS ACCOMPLISHED?	
A	ACHIEVABLE HOW CAN THE GOAL BE ACCOMPLISHED?	
R	RELEVANT DOES THIS SEEM WORTHWHILE?	
T	TIME BOUND WHEN CAN I ACCOMPLISH THIS GOAL?	

SMART

GOALS

WHEN SETTING GOALS, MAKE SURE IT FOLLOWS THE SMART STRUCTURE. USE THE QUESTIONS BELOW TO CREATE YOUR GOALS.

S	SPECIFIC WHAT DO I WANT TO ACCOMPLISH?	
M	MEASURABLE HOW WILL I KNOW WHEN IT IS ACCOMPLISHED?	
A	ACHIEVABLE HOW CAN THE GOAL BE ACCOMPLISHED?	
R	RELEVANT DOES THIS SEEM WORTHWHILE?	
T	TIME BOUND WHEN CAN I ACCOMPLISH THIS GOAL?	

SMART

GOALS

WHEN SETTING GOALS, MAKE SURE IT FOLLOWS THE SMART STRUCTURE. USE THE QUESTIONS BELOW TO CREATE YOUR GOALS.

S	SPECIFIC WHAT DO I WANT TO ACCOMPLISH?	
M	MEASURABLE HOW WILL I KNOW WHEN IT IS ACCOMPLISHED?	
A	ACHIEVABLE HOW CAN THE GOAL BE ACCOMPLISHED?	
R	RELEVANT DOES THIS SEEM WORTHWHILE?	
T	TIME BOUND WHEN CAN I ACCOMPLISH THIS GOAL?	

FILLABLE

CHECKLIST

FILL IN THE CHECKLIST SPACES BELOW WITH SELF-CARE ACTIVITIES THAT YOU CAN DO IN THE MORNING AND AT NIGHT.

MORNING SELF-CARE

- [ ] ______________________________
- [ ] ______________________________
- [ ] ______________________________
- [ ] ______________________________
- [ ] ______________________________
- [ ] ______________________________
- [ ] ______________________________
- [ ] ______________________________

NIGHT SELF-CARE

- [ ] ______________________________
- [ ] ______________________________
- [ ] ______________________________
- [ ] ______________________________
- [ ] ______________________________
- [ ] ______________________________
- [ ] ______________________________
- [ ] ______________________________

FILLABLE

CHECKLIST

FILL IN THE CHECKLIST SPACES BELOW WITH SELF-CARE ACTIVITIES THAT YOU CAN DO IN THE MORNING AND AT NIGHT.

MORNING SELF-CARE

- [ ] ______
- [ ] ______
- [ ] ______
- [ ] ______
- [ ] ______
- [ ] ______
- [ ] ______
- [ ] ______

NIGHT SELF-CARE

- [ ] ______
- [ ] ______
- [ ] ______
- [ ] ______
- [ ] ______
- [ ] ______
- [ ] ______
- [ ] ______

FILLABLE

CHECKLIST

FILL IN THE CHECKLIST SPACES BELOW WITH SELF-CARE ACTIVITIES THAT YOU CAN DO IN THE MORNING AND AT NIGHT.

MORNING SELF-CARE

- [ ] ______________________________
- [ ] ______________________________
- [ ] ______________________________
- [ ] ______________________________
- [ ] ______________________________
- [ ] ______________________________
- [ ] ______________________________
- [ ] ______________________________

NIGHT SELF-CARE

- [ ] ______________________________
- [ ] ______________________________
- [ ] ______________________________
- [ ] ______________________________
- [ ] ______________________________
- [ ] ______________________________
- [ ] ______________________________
- [ ] ______________________________

FILLABLE

CHECKLIST

FILL IN THE CHECKLIST SPACES BELOW WITH SELF-CARE ACTIVITIES THAT YOU CAN DO IN THE MORNING AND AT NIGHT.

MORNING SELF-CARE

- [ ] ______
- [ ] ______
- [ ] ______
- [ ] ______
- [ ] ______
- [ ] ______
- [ ] ______
- [ ] ______

NIGHT SELF-CARE

- [ ] ______
- [ ] ______
- [ ] ______
- [ ] ______
- [ ] ______
- [ ] ______
- [ ] ______
- [ ] ______

WHEEL OF
LIFE

THE WHEEL OF LIFE IS A GREAT TOOL THAT HELPS YOU BETTER UNDERSTAND WHAT YOU CAN DO TO MAKE YOUR LIFE MORE BALANCED. THINK ABOUT THE 8 LIFE CATEGORIES BELOW, AND RATE THEM FROM 1 - 10.

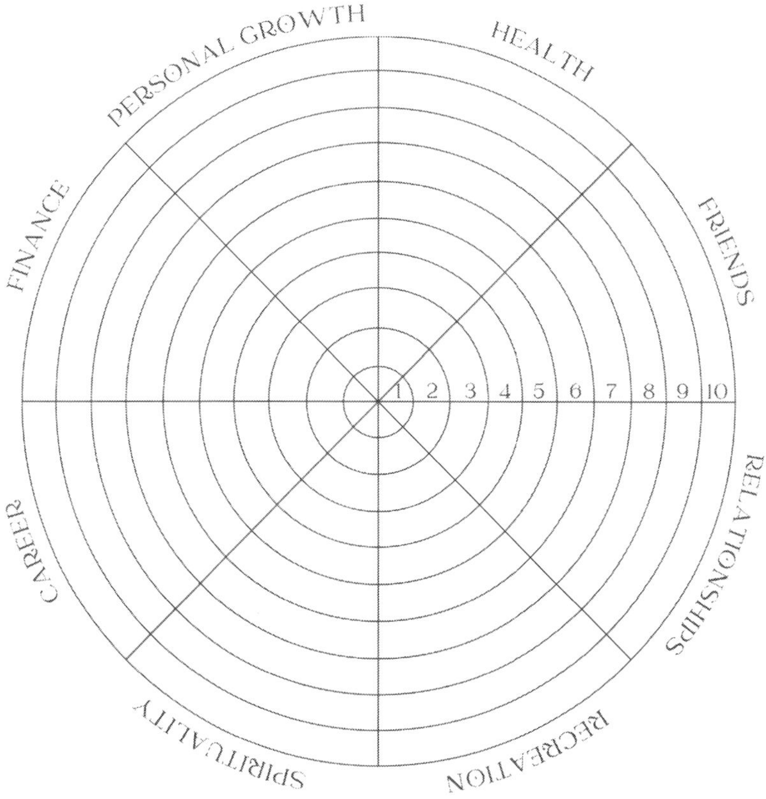

WHEEL OF
LIFE

THE WHEEL OF LIFE IS A GREAT TOOL THAT HELPS YOU BETTER UNDERSTAND WHAT YOU CAN DO TO MAKE YOUR LIFE MORE BALANCED. THINK ABOUT THE 8 LIFE CATEGORIES BELOW, AND RATE THEM FROM 1 - 10.

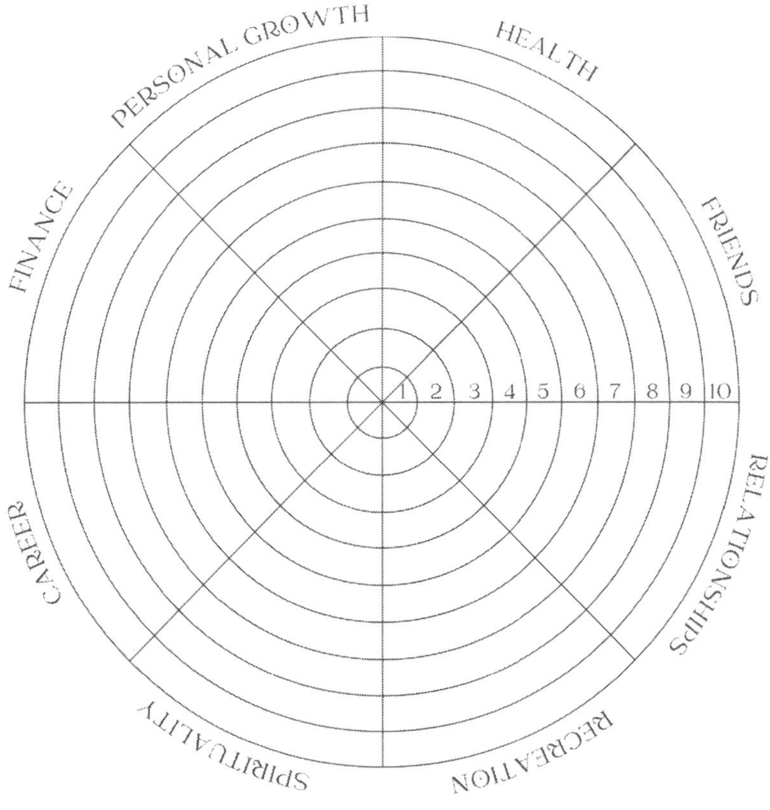

WHEEL OF

LIFE

THE WHEEL OF LIFE IS A GREAT TOOL THAT HELPS YOU BETTER UNDERSTAND WHAT YOU CAN DO TO MAKE YOUR LIFE MORE BALANCED. THINK ABOUT THE 8 LIFE CATEGORIES BELOW, AND RATE THEM FROM 1 - 10.

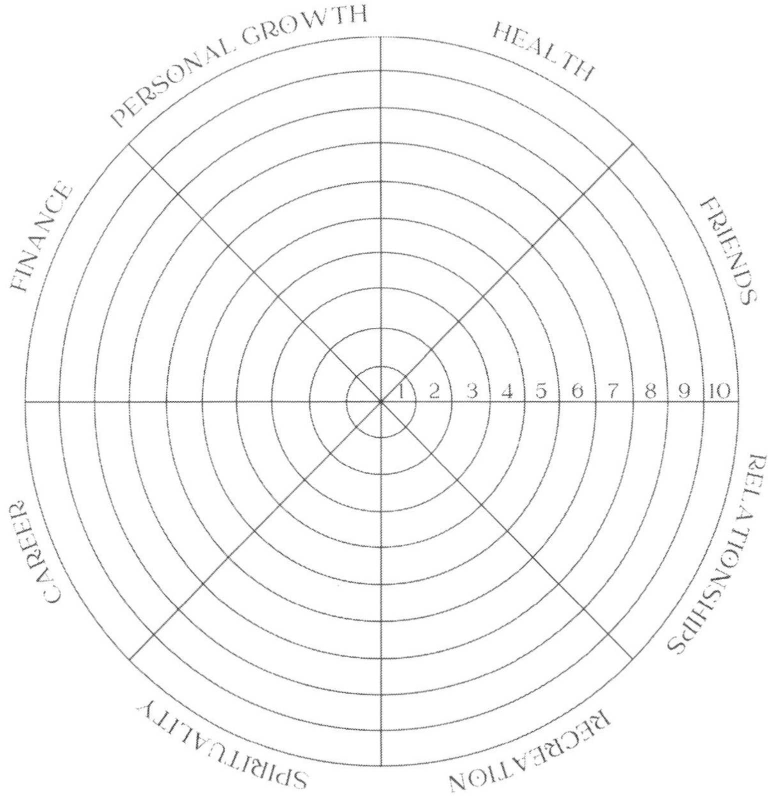

WHEEL OF

LIFE

THE WHEEL OF LIFE IS A GREAT TOOL THAT HELPS YOU BETTER UNDERSTAND WHAT YOU CAN DO TO MAKE YOUR LIFE MORE BALANCED. THINK ABOUT THE 8 LIFE CATEGORIES BELOW, AND RATE THEM FROM 1 - 10.

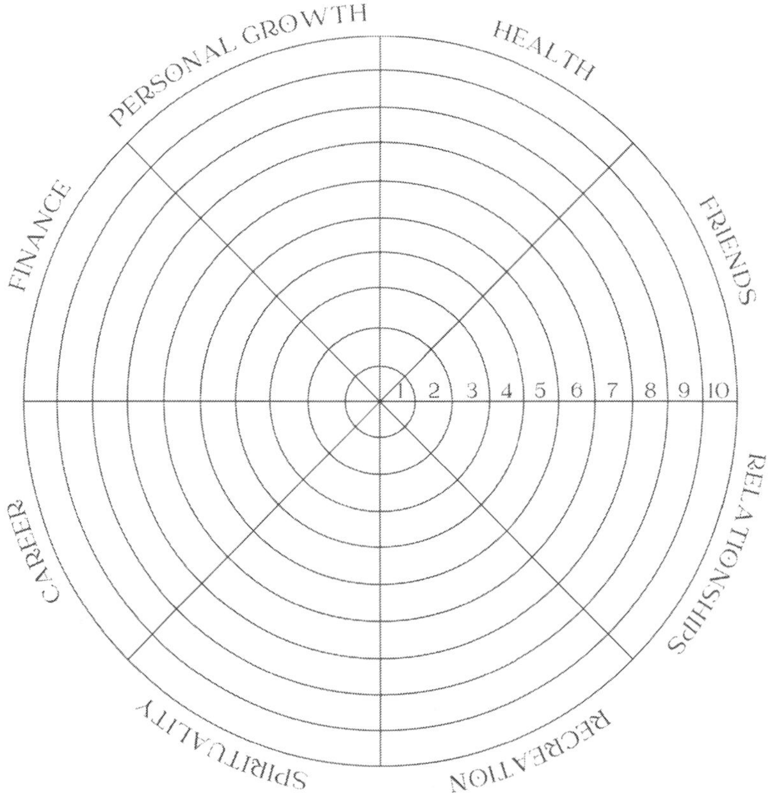

SUCCESS LOG

DAY

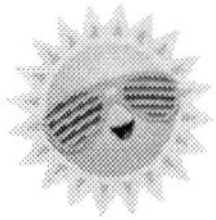

DAILY AFFIRMATIONS

TODAY I AM GRATEFUL FOR

TODAY'S TOP GOALS

01

02

03

SCHEDULE

MOOD

SUCCESS LOG

NIGHT

BREATH

TODAY I AM GRATEFUL FOR

TOP 5 DONE WELL

01

02

03

04

05

DID I COMMUNICATE EFFECTIVELY?

WOULD I DO SOMETHING DIFFERENTLY?

SUCCESS LOG

DAY

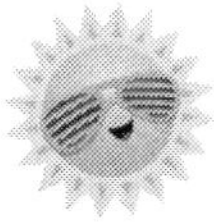

DAILY AFFIRMATIONS

TODAY I AM GRATEFUL FOR

TODAY'S TOP GOALS

01

02

03

SCHEDULE

MOOD

SUCCESS LOG

NIGHT

BREATH

TODAY I AM GRATEFUL FOR

TOP 5 DONE WELL

01

02

03

04

05

DID I COMMUNICATE EFFECTIVELY?

WOULD I DO SOMETHING DIFFERENTLY?

SUCCESS LOG

DAY

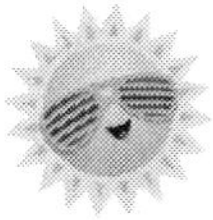

DAILY AFFIRMATIONS

TODAY I AM GRATEFUL FOR

TODAY'S TOP GOALS

01

02

03

SCHEDULE

MOOD

SUCCESS LOG

NIGHT

BREATH

TODAY I AM GRATEFUL FOR

TOP 5 DONE WELL

01

02

03

04

05

DID I COMMUNICATE EFFECTIVELY?

WOULD I DO SOMETHING DIFFERENTLY?

SUCCESS LOG

DAY 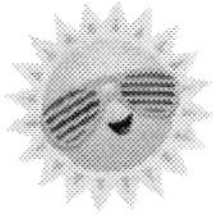

DAILY AFFIRMATIONS

TODAY I AM GRATEFUL FOR

TODAY'S TOP GOALS

01

02

03

SCHEDULE

MOOD

SUCCESS LOG

NIGHT

BREATH

TODAY I AM GRATEFUL FOR

TOP 5 DONE WELL

01

02

03

04

05

DID I COMMUNICATE EFFECTIVELY?

WOULD I DO SOMETHING DIFFERENTLY?

SUCCESS LOG

DAY

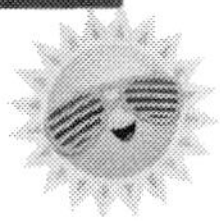

DAILY AFFIRMATIONS

TODAY I AM GRATEFUL FOR

TODAY'S TOP GOALS

01

02

03

SCHEDULE

MOOD

SUCCESS LOG

NIGHT

BREATH

TODAY I AM GRATEFUL FOR

TOP 5 DONE WELL

01

02

03

04

05

DID I COMMUNICATE EFFECTIVELY?

WOULD I DO SOMETHING DIFFERENTLY?

SUCCESS LOG

DAY

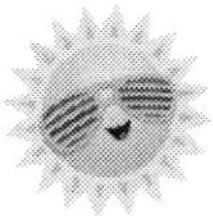

DAILY AFFIRMATIONS

TODAY I AM GRATEFUL FOR

TODAY'S TOP GOALS

01

02

03

SCHEDULE

MOOD

SUCCESS LOG

NIGHT

BREATH

TODAY I AM GRATEFUL FOR

TOP 5 DONE WELL

01

02

03

04

05

DID I COMMUNICATE EFFECTIVELY?

WOULD I DO SOMETHING DIFFERENTLY?

SUCCESS LOG

DAY

DAILY AFFIRMATIONS

TODAY I AM GRATEFUL FOR

TODAY'S TOP GOALS

01

02

03

SCHEDULE

MOOD

SUCCESS LOG

NIGHT

BREATH

TODAY I AM GRATEFUL FOR

TOP 5 DONE WELL

01

02

03

04

05

DID I COMMUNICATE EFFECTIVELY?

WOULD I DO SOMETHING DIFFERENTLY?

SUCCESS LOG

DAY

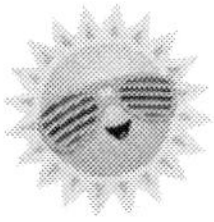

DAILY AFFIRMATIONS

TODAY I AM GRATEFUL FOR

TODAY'S TOP GOALS

01

02

03

SCHEDULE

MOOD

SUCCESS LOG

NIGHT

BREATH

TODAY I AM GRATEFUL FOR

TOP 5 DONE WELL

01

02

03

04

05

DID I COMMUNICATE EFFECTIVELY?

WOULD I DO SOMETHING DIFFERENTLY?

SUCCESS LOG

DAY

DAILY AFFIRMATIONS

TODAY I AM GRATEFUL FOR

TODAY'S TOP GOALS

01

02

03

SCHEDULE

MOOD

SUCCESS LOG

NIGHT

BREATH

TODAY I AM GRATEFUL FOR

TOP 5 DONE WELL

01

02

03

04

05

DID I COMMUNICATE EFFECTIVELY?

WOULD I DO SOMETHING DIFFERENTLY?

SUCCESS LOG

DAY

DAILY AFFIRMATIONS

TODAY I AM GRATEFUL FOR

TODAY'S TOP GOALS

01

02

03

SCHEDULE

MOOD

SUCCESS LOG

NIGHT

BREATH

TODAY I AM GRATEFUL FOR

TOP 5 DONE WELL

01

02

03

04

05

DID I COMMUNICATE EFFECTIVELY?

WOULD I DO SOMETHING DIFFERENTLY?

SUCCESS LOG

DAY

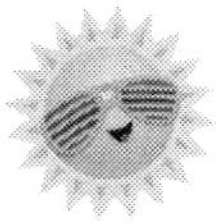

DAILY AFFIRMATIONS

TODAY I AM GRATEFUL FOR

TODAY'S TOP GOALS

01

02

03

SCHEDULE

MOOD

SUCCESS LOG

NIGHT

BREATH

TODAY I AM GRATEFUL FOR

TOP 5 DONE WELL

01

02

03

04

05

DID I COMMUNICATE EFFECTIVELY?

WOULD I DO SOMETHING DIFFERENTLY?

SUCCESS LOG

DAY

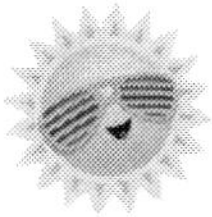

DAILY AFFIRMATIONS

TODAY I AM GRATEFUL FOR

TODAY'S TOP GOALS

01

02

03

SCHEDULE

MOOD

SUCCESS LOG

NIGHT

BREATH

TODAY I AM GRATEFUL FOR

TOP 5 DONE WELL

01

02

03

04

05

DID I COMMUNICATE EFFECTIVELY?

WOULD I DO SOMETHING DIFFERENTLY?

SUCCESS LOG

DAY

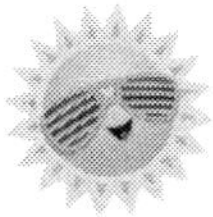

DAILY AFFIRMATIONS

TODAY I AM GRATEFUL FOR

TODAY'S TOP GOALS

01

02

03

SCHEDULE

MOOD

SUCCESS LOG

NIGHT

BREATH

TODAY I AM GRATEFUL FOR

TOP 5 DONE WELL

01

02

03

04

05

DID I COMMUNICATE EFFECTIVELY?

WOULD I DO SOMETHING DIFFERENTLY?

SUCCESS LOG

DAY

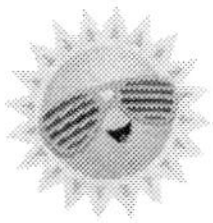

DAILY AFFIRMATIONS

TODAY I AM GRATEFUL FOR

TODAY'S TOP GOALS

01

02

03

SCHEDULE

MOOD

SUCCESS LOG

NIGHT

BREATH

TODAY I AM GRATEFUL FOR

TOP 5 DONE WELL

01

02

03

04

05

DID I COMMUNICATE EFFECTIVELY?

WOULD I DO SOMETHING DIFFERENTLY?

SUCCESS LOG

DAY

DAILY AFFIRMATIONS

TODAY I AM GRATEFUL FOR

TODAY'S TOP GOALS

01

02

03

SCHEDULE

MOOD

SUCCESS LOG

NIGHT

BREATH

TODAY I AM GRATEFUL FOR

TOP 5 DONE WELL

01

02

03

04

05

DID I COMMUNICATE EFFECTIVELY?

WOULD I DO SOMETHING DIFFERENTLY?

SUCCESS LOG

DAY

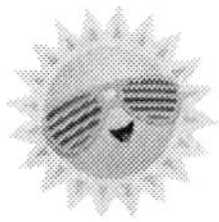

DAILY AFFIRMATIONS

TODAY I AM GRATEFUL FOR

TODAY'S TOP GOALS

01

02

03

SCHEDULE

MOOD

SUCCESS LOG

NIGHT

BREATH

TODAY I AM GRATEFUL FOR

TOP 5 DONE WELL

01

02

03

04

05

DID I COMMUNICATE EFFECTIVELY?

WOULD I DO SOMETHING DIFFERENTLY?

SUCCESS LOG

DAY

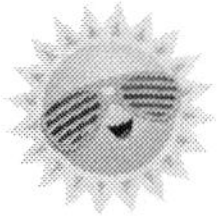

DAILY AFFIRMATIONS

TODAY I AM GRATEFUL FOR

TODAY'S TOP GOALS

01

02

03

SCHEDULE

MOOD

SUCCESS LOG

NIGHT

BREATH

TODAY I AM GRATEFUL FOR

TOP 5 DONE WELL

01

02

03

04

05

DID I COMMUNICATE EFFECTIVELY?

WOULD I DO SOMETHING DIFFERENTLY?

SUCCESS LOG

DAY

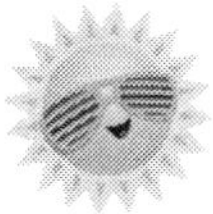

DAILY AFFIRMATIONS

TODAY I AM GRATEFUL FOR

TODAY'S TOP GOALS

01

02

03

SCHEDULE

MOOD

SUCCESS LOG

NIGHT

BREATH

TODAY I AM GRATEFUL FOR

TOP 5 DONE WELL

01

02

03

04

05

DID I COMMUNICATE EFFECTIVELY?

WOULD I DO SOMETHING DIFFERENTLY?

SUCCESS LOG

DAY

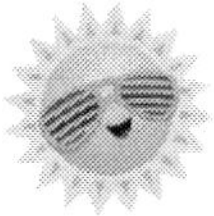

DAILY AFFIRMATIONS

TODAY I AM GRATEFUL FOR

TODAY'S TOP GOALS

01

02

03

SCHEDULE

MOOD

SUCCESS LOG

NIGHT

BREATH

TODAY I AM GRATEFUL FOR

TOP 5 DONE WELL

01

02

03

04

05

DID I COMMUNICATE EFFECTIVELY?

WOULD I DO SOMETHING DIFFERENTLY?

SUCCESS LOG

DAY

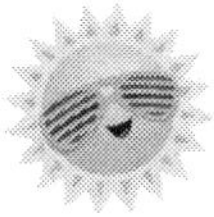

DAILY AFFIRMATIONS

TODAY I AM GRATEFUL FOR

TODAY'S TOP GOALS

01

02

03

SCHEDULE

MOOD

SUCCESS LOG

NIGHT

BREATH

TODAY I AM GRATEFUL FOR

TOP 5 DONE WELL

01

02

03

04

05

DID I COMMUNICATE EFFECTIVELY?

WOULD I DO SOMETHING DIFFERENTLY?

SUCCESS LOG

DAY

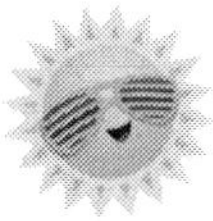

DAILY AFFIRMATIONS

TODAY I AM GRATEFUL FOR

TODAY'S TOP GOALS

01

02

03

SCHEDULE

MOOD

SUCCESS LOG

NIGHT

BREATH

TODAY I AM GRATEFUL FOR

TOP 5 DONE WELL

01

02

03

04

05

DID I COMMUNICATE EFFECTIVELY?

WOULD I DO SOMETHING DIFFERENTLY?

SUCCESS LOG

DAY

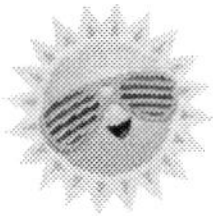

DAILY AFFIRMATIONS

TODAY I AM GRATEFUL FOR

TODAY'S TOP GOALS

01

02

03

SCHEDULE

MOOD

SUCCESS LOG

NIGHT

BREATH

TODAY I AM GRATEFUL FOR

TOP 5 DONE WELL

01

02

03

04

05

DID I COMMUNICATE EFFECTIVELY?

WOULD I DO SOMETHING DIFFERENTLY?

SUCCESS LOG

DAY

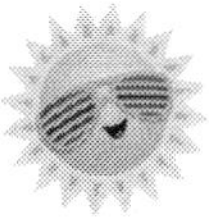

DAILY AFFIRMATIONS

TODAY I AM GRATEFUL FOR

TODAY'S TOP GOALS

01

02

03

SCHEDULE

MOOD

SUCCESS LOG

NIGHT

BREATH

TODAY I AM GRATEFUL FOR

TOP 5 DONE WELL

01

02

03

04

05

DID I COMMUNICATE EFFECTIVELY?

WOULD I DO SOMETHING DIFFERENTLY?

SUCCESS LOG

DAY

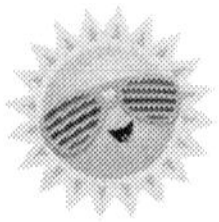

DAILY AFFIRMATIONS

TODAY I AM GRATEFUL FOR

TODAY'S TOP GOALS

01

02

03

SCHEDULE

MOOD

SUCCESS LOG

NIGHT

BREATH

TODAY I AM GRATEFUL FOR

TOP 5 DONE WELL

01

02

03

04

05

DID I COMMUNICATE EFFECTIVELY?

WOULD I DO SOMETHING DIFFERENTLY?

SUCCESS LOG

DAY

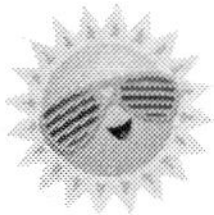

DAILY AFFIRMATIONS

TODAY I AM GRATEFUL FOR

TODAY'S TOP GOALS

01

02

03

SCHEDULE

MOOD

SUCCESS LOG

NIGHT

BREATH

TODAY I AM GRATEFUL FOR

TOP 5 DONE WELL

01

02

03

04

05

DID I COMMUNICATE EFFECTIVELY?

WOULD I DO SOMETHING DIFFERENTLY?

SUCCESS LOG

DAY

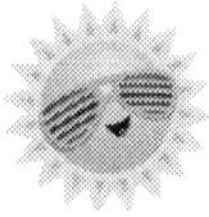

DAILY AFFIRMATIONS

TODAY I AM GRATEFUL FOR

TODAY'S TOP GOALS

01

02

03

SCHEDULE

MOOD

SUCCESS LOG

NIGHT

BREATH

TODAY I AM GRATEFUL FOR

TOP 5 DONE WELL

01

02

03

04

05

DID I COMMUNICATE EFFECTIVELY?

WOULD I DO SOMETHING DIFFERENTLY?

SUCCESS LOG

DAY

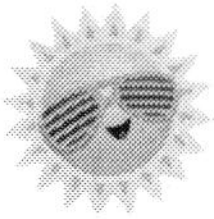

DAILY AFFIRMATIONS

TODAY I AM GRATEFUL FOR

TODAY'S TOP GOALS

01

02

03

SCHEDULE

MOOD

SUCCESS LOG

NIGHT

BREATH

TODAY I AM GRATEFUL FOR

TOP 5 DONE WELL

01

02

03

04

05

DID I COMMUNICATE EFFECTIVELY?

WOULD I DO SOMETHING DIFFERENTLY?

SUCCESS LOG

DAY

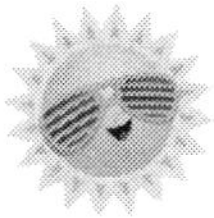

DAILY AFFIRMATIONS

TODAY I AM GRATEFUL FOR

TODAY'S TOP GOALS

01

02

03

SCHEDULE

MOOD

SUCCESS LOG

NIGHT

BREATH

TODAY I AM GRATEFUL FOR

TOP 5 DONE WELL

01

02

03

04

05

DID I COMMUNICATE EFFECTIVELY?

WOULD I DO SOMETHING DIFFERENTLY?

ACTION PRIORITY

MATRIX

THE ACTION PRIORITY MATRIX IS A GREAT WAY TO VISUALISE WHAT TASKS TAKE PRIORITY OVER OTHERS, AND HOW TO BEST ALLOCATE YOUR TIME TOWARDS THEM.

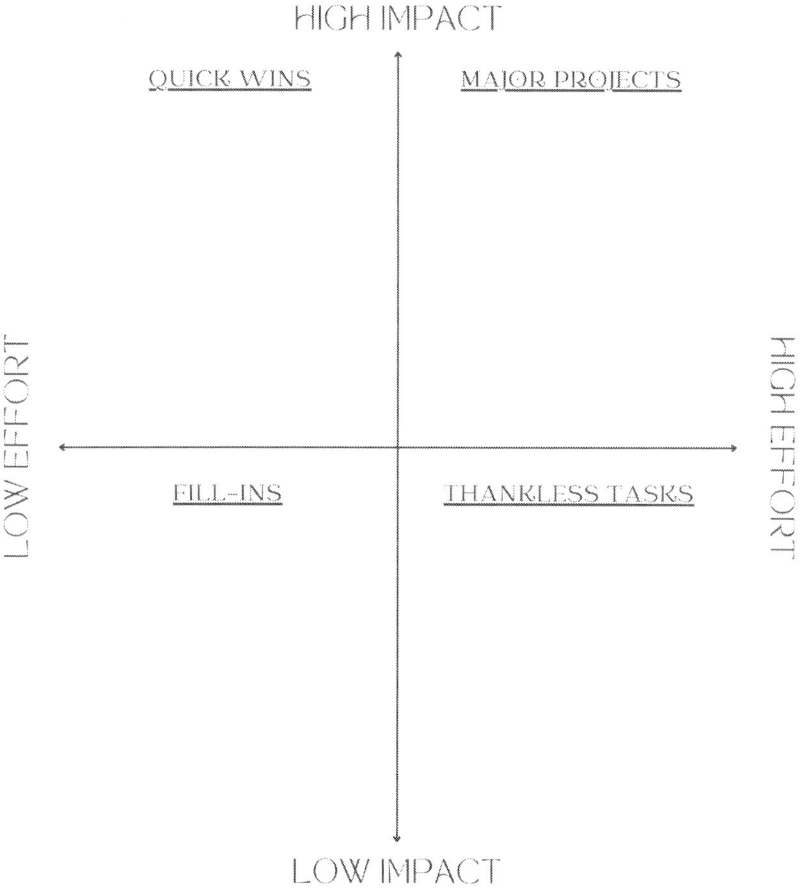

ACTION PRIORITY

MATRIX

THE ACTION PRIORITY MATRIX IS A GREAT WAY TO VISUALISE WHAT TASKS TAKE PRIORITY OVER OTHERS, AND HOW TO BEST ALLOCATE YOUR TIME TOWARDS THEM.

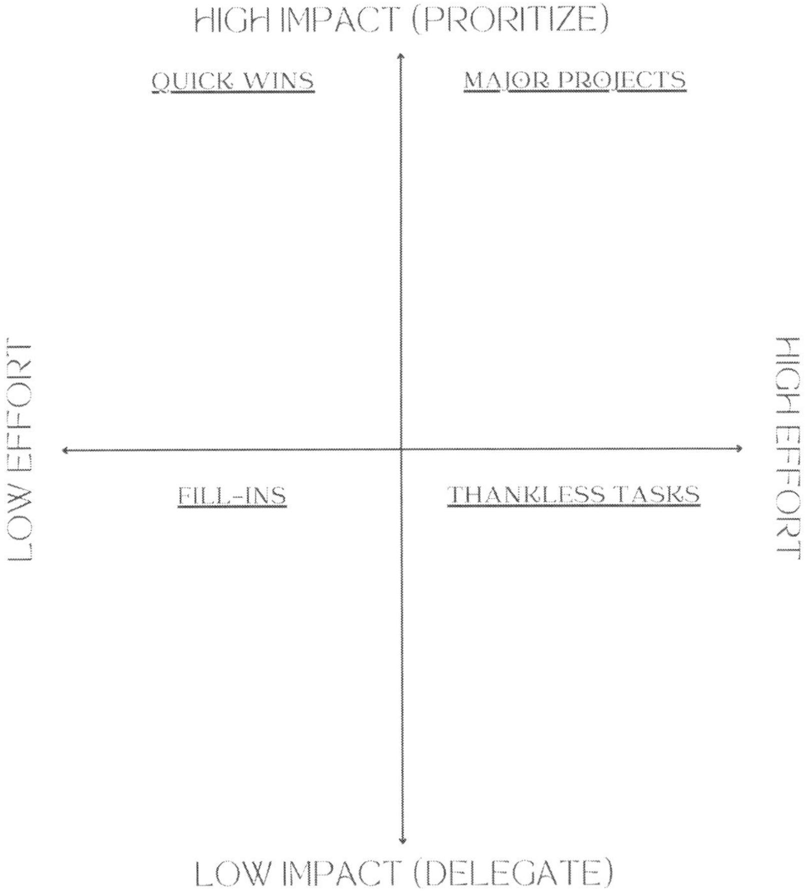

ACTION PRIORITY

MATRIX

THE ACTION PRIORITY MATRIX IS A GREAT WAY TO VISUALISE WHAT TASKS TAKE PRIORITY OVER OTHERS, AND HOW TO BEST ALLOCATE YOUR TIME TOWARDS THEM.

HIGH IMPACT (PRORITIZE)

QUICK WINS

MAJOR PROJECTS

LOW EFFORT

HIGH EFFORT

FILL-INS

THANKLESS TASKS

LOW IMPACT (DELEGATE)

ACTION PRIORITY

MATRIX

THE ACTION PRIORITY MATRIX IS A GREAT WAY TO VISUALISE WHAT TASKS TAKE PRIORITY OVER OTHERS, AND HOW TO BEST ALLOCATE YOUR TIME TOWARDS THEM.

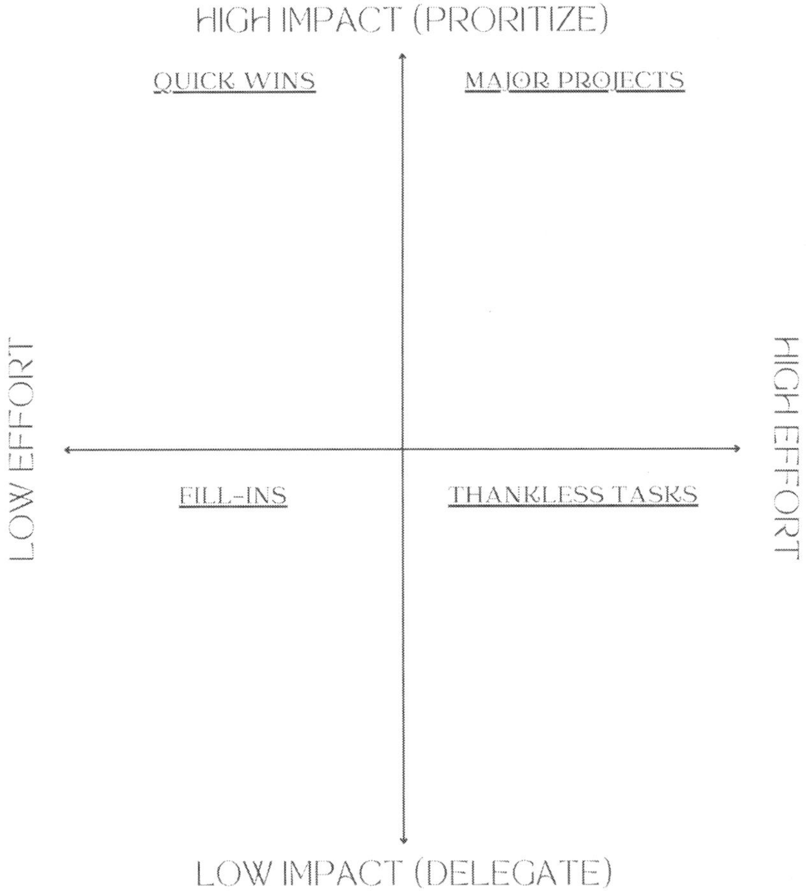

ACTION PRIORITY

MATRIX

THE ACTION PRIORITY MATRIX IS A GREAT WAY TO VISUALISE WHAT TASKS TAKE PRIORITY OVER OTHERS, AND HOW TO BEST ALLOCATE YOUR TIME TOWARDS THEM.

HIGH IMPACT (PRORITIZE)

QUICK WINS

MAJOR PROJECTS

LOW EFFORT

HIGH EFFORT

FILL-INS

THANKLESS TASKS

LOW IMPACT (DELEGATE)

THANK YOU

THANK YOU FOR SUPPORTING OUR BUSINESS.

LEAVE US A REVIEW AND LET OTHERS KNOW WHAT YOU THINK!!

CHECK OUT OUR OTHER WORKBOOKS

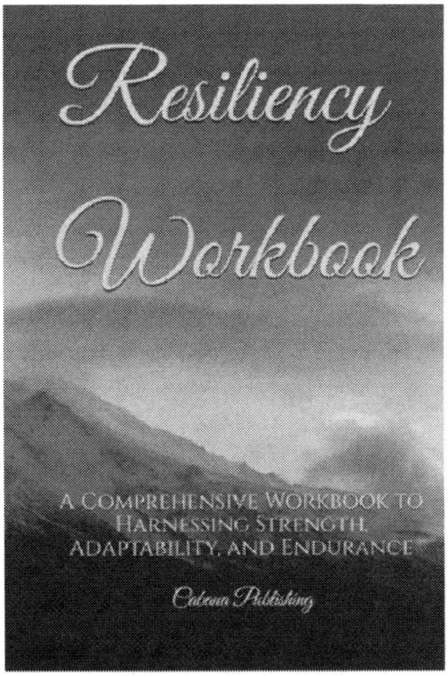

WWW.CABANA.MEDIA

Made in the USA
Monee, IL
11 November 2026

af5cb09a-db6f-4c59-a7c6-6dcd2e862105R01